Helpful Beauty Remedies
By Shirley Cross

This book is dedicated to my daughter S.D. Cross and A. Cross with love.

About the author:

Samm Cross has spent 30 plus years in the beauty industry as a cosmetologist.
People love simple yet effective beauty ideas to help their day go easier. These tips are tried and time tested by countless women to help improve their beauty regimen.

This book was put together for a simple helpful place to get ideas that make our beauty regimen easier with some natural remedies. These simple but wonderful products that most people have at home can substitute in an emergency and are often a healthier alternative to complex chemical laden products. Often when we are not careful what we use on our bodies or hair problems arise. Toxins can easily build up from prolong use. Hopefully, there are some tips that will make your day easier and more beautiful!

For longer thicker lashes and brows

This works as well as some of the more expensive eyelash products and it's healthy for your body as well.

Wash an old mascara or a small container and fill with equal amounts of Castor Oil, Vitamin E Oil and a drop of olive oil. Mix the concoction together as well as you can with your mascara wand, and apply a light layer to lashes (or brows) every night before bed. Castor oil thickens your lashes and Vitamin E and olive oil accelerates growth. Give it 4 months or so for best results.

For longer thicker looking lashes using mascara start by putting a coat of powder on the lashes, baby powder or face powder is fine. Follow this with a volumizing mascara, next use a lengthening mascara and end with a waterproof mascara to lightly sweep over the tips and

corner of your lashes to finish the look.

Winged or cat eye look

Use a plastic knife, business card or tape to help you draw a straight line. This makes the process much easier. The plastic knife is the most economical because you can wipe it off and reuse for a longer period of time this will save money. Start at the corner of the eye draw your line, next the center going towards the outer corner, then the inner corner of the eye. Drawing the line in separate parts makes it easier to get a straight line.

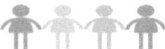

Cellulite wrap

Coffee and Coconut Oil Scrub:

1/2 cup ground Coffee, 1 cup Olive or Coconut oil. Coffee is the wonder ingredient in this antioxidant packed-scrub: it not only reinvigorates your senses, but it also lightens and brightens the skin this temporarily minimizes cellulite. Pair it with creamy coconut oil is one of the most moisturizing natural ingredients around. Olive oil has been used for centuries to massage and moisturizes skin. Apply generously to problem areas then wrap in saran wrap for 45 minutes, wash off thoroughly.

Homemade body wrap to improve the appearance of cellulite. This will help improve the texture including tightening. Detoxification, rejuvenation, healing and weight loss. Help trim inches off stomach, buttocks, and thighs. To be effective body wraps should be done regularly. Making home wraps are not difficult. There are many this is just one. Fine the best one that works for you. This is a great one to start with.

1/4 cup of sea salt
2 tbsp of olive oil or coconut oil
2 cups of water

1 tsp of your favorite essential oil (lavender) is my favorite
1 cup of herbal powder your favorite (St Johns wort)

boil water, remove from heat, add sea salt let it dissolve. Add the other ingredients and stir to a paste. Let it cool, apply to your body then wrap with plastic wrap, towels or sheet. Leave on for an hour. Stay in an area where you will create the least amount of mess, relax by laying down if possible on the couch, floor or tub. It's usually too messy for the bed. You are home, so make your own choice. There are so many herbs and oils that you can combine for effective wraps just do a little research to find the ones you like the best.

Face cleansing with oil for a softer clearer complexion.

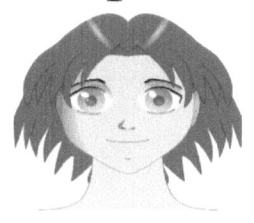

A list of oils that work great, but do your research to find which oil works best for your skin type. Always chose cold-pressed, unprocessed, virgin oils whenever possible.

Avocado oil is good for all skin types, dry and sensitive.

Grape seed oil: for all skin types acne prone, oily normal and sensitive.

Jojoba oil: for all skin types, dry and normal.

Coconut oil: for all skin types: normal, sensitive, dry and acne.

Olive oil: for all skin types normal, oily, sensitive and acne.

Massage in wipe clean with a cloth or tissue and rinse with warm water. Proceed with your usual face routine. Using an oil cleansing routine will help your skin balance it's natural oil production. As always do your research to find what works best for your skin type.

Healthy hair home remedies

Herbal rinses and sprays made with rosemary tea.
Make a tea from the herb and put in a spray bottle
for daily use to mist the hair before styling or in a
squirt bottle to use before conditioning in the
shower. Rosemary tea will help stimulate hair
growth, circulation, moisturize, and much more.
This is an excellent hair tonic.

Aloe Vera juice for moisturizing and closing the cuticle to increase shine. Use as a rinse in the shower or in a spray bottle for everyday use to moisturize.

Green tea has been shown to increase dermal papilla cell to boost hair production along with its antioxidants properties, used in a spray bottle for daily mist to moisturize or in a squirt bottle in the shower as a leave in conditioner.

Essential oils for healthy hair

Here is a list of oils that work wonders on the hair, but feel free to explore ones that you like the best. These can be used daily to massage in or as oil treatments before washing the hair it depends on your hair and personal preference. Use a small amount for daily use and a generous amount for oil treatment to massage into the scalp and hair before washing the hair.

Always chose cold-pressed, unprocessed, virgin oils whenever possible.

Coconut oil, Jojoba oil

Olive oil, Sweet almond oil

Grapeseed oil, Avocado oil

Caster oil, Tea tree oil

Emu oil, Argan oil, peppermint oil, just to name a few but there are so many more.

These are a list of a few key Vitamins and supplements that promote hair growth. Of course, all vitamins are an important part of any cell growth, these are most helpful. Try to get them from a fresh food source whenever possible but supplements also work well and in conjunction with a nutritious food source.

Protein, Collagen, Silica, vitamin C, A,B complex,

Biotin, Alpha-Lipoic acid, Lutein, D3, Pantothenic acid.

For cleaning and removing buildup from your hair try, a solution of baking soda diluted in water to make it easier to saturate the hair, followed by apple cider vinegar diluted with equal parts water. Use a squeeze bottle for easier application of baking soda and vinegar solution on hair. Massage and squeeze this through the hair thoroughly then rinse until the water runs clear. Use baking soda with caution, because using it to often can dry out the hair. Finish by adding some extra virgin coconut oil, adjust the amount to accommodate your hair texture. This should make your hair clean, shiny and very soft. Pay attention to the condition of your hair, a deep cleanse usually isn't necessary more than once a month. If you have color or keratin treatments on your hair a deep cleanse might remove some of your product, so consider this carefully before you proceed.

For your healthiest hair and optimum hair length

retention and growth, use heatless hairstyles whenever possible. Roller sets, twists outs, braids, braid outs, buns, ponytails, Bantu knots, pipe cleaners, curl formers, or your favorite way to avoid the stress of heat on your hair daily.

Growth occurs a half an inch per month on average, an inch or more growth can happen, but this is not usual for most and is fast growth.

Learn to give your hair love and attention, this will help improve your overall hair health and appearance.

Remembering that moisture comes from water, but can be enhanced with the right moisturizing products. Aloe Vera, Caster oil, coconut oil and honey are just a few.

Use apple cider vinegar to detangle and prevent dandruff.

Use mascara or your face powder to cover gray on hairline and parts in between color touch-ups. This lessens the use of hair color for healthier hair.

 Use an egg to make a protein mask for shiny hair.

Achieve hair growth retention for longer hair with this super powerful hair mask using natural ingredients! Increase or decrease according to the amount of hair you have, this is a general guideline.

Most of these items can be found in your kitchen.

Items needed for this mask…

1 egg
1 tbsp. Mashed Banana
1 tbsp. Mashed Avocado
1 tbsp. Plain Greek Yogurt
1 tbsp. Almond Milk
1 tbsp. Coconut Milk

Directions:
Blend together and apply directly to hair. Comb through using your fingers and apply from scalp to ends.

Place hair in a shower cap or plastic and relax for around 20 minutes. You can combine all or two or more of these ingredients to make a powerful mask, which ever ingredients that you have available that's on this list. Remember there are many more healthy choices, you just need to do a little research.

Rinse with cold water and repeat this once a week or alternate ingredients.

Biotin helps strengthen hair and prevent breakage.

Vitamin A is an antioxidant that helps with cell growth and healthy sebum in the scalp.

Zinc helps hair growth and repairs damaged hair.

Iron keeps your hair follicles healthy and scalp oil circulating.

Potassium keeps scalp healthy and helps prevent hair loss.

Vitamin C helps keep your hair strong and rich in color.

Treating your hair with protein conditioners can help improve the structure of the hair and more moisturized, leaving the hair softer less likely to break.

Onion juice can help stimulate hair growth and get rid of Alopecia. Onion's high sulfur content helps boost collagen production, there promoting hair growth. Just boil an onion let it cool, strain it and use the juice as a hair treatment, leave on twenty minutes. Rinse and use your normal conditioner to finish your process. Use every two weeks at least until desired growth, thereafter use once a month.

Apple cider vinegar rinse helps maintain the PH balance of the hair, this helps with hair growth.

Henna, when used regularly, will make the hair

thicker and shinier by coating and lay down the cuticle of the hair. It will build up over time making a thicker strand of hair. This works great for people with fine hair, just use once a month.

Stretch mark remedy

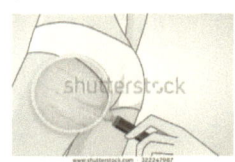

Cocoa Butter

- Cocoa butter treats very well the stretch marks and is also very good at preventing them from appearing. Apply cocoa butter once a day on the affected areas and you will notice the healing process and the result. You will have less visible stretch marks with less effort.

Aloe Vera

- By applying Aloe Vera gel every morning on your stretch marks you will see amazing results: the stretch marks will slowly start to fade. Aloe Vera is one of the most commonly used home treatment with highly healing properties.

Vitamin E

- Like in many other cases, home-made remedies can greatly vary from one person to other. Vitamin E is one of the remedies that many women say it has magical results. All you need to do is to apply daily on your affected areas and the stretch marks will gradually start to fade. You can also use soap with Vitamin E and it will have the same effect.

Lavender Oil

- It is really difficult to make the stretch marks disappear, but you can at least make them less noticeable. Lavender oil is also one of the most used and known remedies for stretch marks. You need to apply three times a day on the stretch marks and it will make them less visible. It is very cheap and if applied properly, you will see some improvements to your skin.

Your own secret blend

- You can create a paste from mixing Vitamin E with half a cup of olive oil and a quarter of a cup of Aloe Vera. This home-made remedy is very efficient for both treatment and prevention of the stretch marks.

Camphor and mint oils also work great because they increase circulation. Be careful with these two because they can cause a burning sensation on sensitive skin. These are some of the most effective home remedies to help heal and eliminate stretch marks. One thing to remember is to be consistent! If you don't do anything they are going to stay, with some persistence you will see a marked improvement and for some, they will heal completely. Like most things in life, the effort you put in is what you will get out. A major benefit of this massage also is softer and smoother skin.

Treatment For Acne

Some helpful home remedies for acne

If you are suffering from painful cystic acne and need a quick remedy these will help.

1: camphor oil does wonder almost an overnight relief. There are several products that are sold in stores for colds and decongest that can be used. Just wash your face and apply before bed, be careful and keep away from the eyes and mouth or any other sensitive areas because camphor can cause a burning sensation. Wash your hands after applying or use a Q-tip.

2: lemon juice and baking soda mixed into a paste and applied to the affected area after washing the face and left overnight will help dry up the acne. As with any product that can burn keep this away from the eyes or any sensitive areas.

3: toothpaste can be applied to the acne which will help dry them, wash your face then dab toothpaste on affected areas leave overnight. As with any product that can cause a burn so keep this away from the eyes or any sensitive areas.

4: activated charcoal and bentonite clay a tea spoon each mixed into a paste and applied to the face and let dry for 20 minutes. Avoid getting too close to the eyes.

Bald Spot Hair Regrowth

If you are suffering from thinning or balding hair or edges due to hormonal, nerve damage or abuse, these natural remedies are known to help regrow your hair.

First of all, be patience, because only time can guarantee regrowth. Keep your hair clean by washing at least once a week. Massage oil into the scalp thoroughly and cover with a plastic cap for 10 to 20 minutes before shampooing.

Now there are oils that can also help.

1. Emu oil has an excellent reputation for helping hair regrow in trouble spots.

2. Caster oil is another wonderful oil for hair regrowth. Caster oil moisturize, soften, hydrates and seals in moisture.

3. Coconut, Grapeseed, Olive, are a few of the easily accessible natural oils that are known to improve hair growth. Many others are available so you can make your own choice.

4. Rosemary and nettle tea used in a spray bottle to spritz hair several times a week. Improves circulation and helps to heal any damage to the scalp.

After you wash your hair and towel dry it apply a small amount of either oil to the problem area and massage for a few minutes.

If your hair is naturally oily you can use the oil before you shampoo. Use a few times a week if you don't have a problem with using oil in your hair.

It takes three to six months to see a significance amount of hair growth, be patient it will happen.

Whatever you were doing to get the damaged hair discontinue if you want to retain your new growth. Do special treatments with protein and deep conditioners. Moisturize and use leave in conditioners for hair that is dry or brittle.

RECONSTRUCTOR CONDITIONERS

NEVER UNDERESTIMATE RECONSTRUCTOR AND DEEP CONDITIONERS TO HELP REPAIR AND RESTORE THE STRENGTH AND HEALTH OF YOUR HAIR.

SO OFTEN WE AS WOMEN IN GENERAL ABUSE OUR HAIR, ON A DAILY BASIS, BUT FORGET OR NEGLECT TO ATTEMPT ANY REPAIR OF OUR HAIR HEALTH.

MOST PEOPLE USE A basic CONDITIONER BUT usually DON'T TAKE EXTRA TIME FOR A

RESTORATIVE CONDITIONER, FOR SEVERAL REASONS WHETHER IT'S TIME, MONEY, OR LACK OF KNOWLEDGE.

WE OFTEN NOTICE BREAKAGE, DULLNESS, LIFELESS OR THINNING BUT   FAIL TO DO ANY REPAIR.

THERE ARE SO MANY GREAT CONDITIONERS ON THE MARKET SO I'M NOT GOING TO USE AND BRAND NAMES BUT JUST FIND ONE THAT SUITS YOUR TYPE OF HAIR BEST.

HOMEMADE ONES WORK JUST AS WELL

ALOE VERA GEL

EGGS

MILK AND HONEY

OLIVE OIL

THESE ARE A FEW OF THE NATURAL CONDITIONERS THAT CAN BE USED TO REPAIR YOUR HAIR.

JUST DO YOUR RESEARCH TO FIND WHAT WORKS BEST FOR YOUR HAIR TYPE. ALLOW AT LEAST 20 MINUTES FOR THE CONDITIONER TO REPAIR THE HAIR. A HOODED DRYER IS BEST BUT YOU CAN PUT A PLASTIC CAP ON AND ALLOW ROOM TEMPRETURE TO HELP THE CONDITIONER TO PENETRATE THE HAIR.

Rinse well using warm or cool water is best.

For a fresh healthy complexion

Start by cleansing with your favorite natural oil. Coconut and vitamin E oil mixed and massaged into the face and wipe off with tissue. Then follow this with your favorite cleanser. Black soap is a great one, because it removes dirt and lightens blemishes as well. Follow this with fresh Aloe Vera gel. Allow to dry then wipe off with a damp cloth. Always put sunscreen to protect from sun damage before you begin your day, makeup or not, this is one of your best defense to keep your skin fresh looking and glowing.